End Knee Pain Forever!

The Truth, the Whole Truth and Nothing but the Truth

By

Dr. J. L. Selano DC CME

If you would like to come to our clinic in
Centennial, CO we are located at:

6726 S. Revere Pkwy STE 180 Centennial, CO 80112. Come in for your no cost, risk free consultation to find out if you are truly a candidate for this incredible procedure.

Please call us at 720-681-6170 to book your initial appointment or visit our website at www.advregenmed.com

Disclaimer

The information provided in this **book** is designed to provide helpful information on the subjects discussed. This **book** is not meant to be used, nor should it be used, to diagnose or treat any **medical** condition. For diagnosis or treatment of any **medical** problem, consult your own physician.

Contents

Foreword

I met Dr. Selano during an interview for his medical director position. He spoke with me only a little while, and we shared more about who we were, rather than what he wanted me to do. He is just like that—honest, caring, and down to earth.

I have spent the greater part of my life either treating folks with addiction or helping those who have taken on the challenge of recovery and found a wonderful new life. The most disheartening thing I have ever seen is patients who treat the symptoms of their illnesses with opiates and, at times, benzodiazepines (drugs like Ativan and Xanax). I watched how these drugs ask for themselves and escalate into a full-fledged addiction or dependence. A majority of pain that patients who take long-term opiates experience is from opiate-induced pain. Dr. Selano agreed that there had to be a better way and introduced me to the wonderful work he is doing.

I have gotten to know him as a voracious businessman who just does not know the word fail. I have seen him combine this voracity with his love of treating patients to develop a system that really works in healing painful conditions that Western medicine would have moving right to surgery or drugs. I have met and worked with our patients, who have found relief and, in many cases, a whole new way of experiencing life without pain.

Dr. Selano has put together an easily readable book that answers and supports all the treatments we employ to do this. To date, no one has done this, even those who do similar work. My wish is that, in reading this, you will find the knowledge and information you need to help dispel misinformation, rumors, myths, and propaganda that some put out about treatments to protect themselves and their pocketbooks.

I am proud and grateful to know him and be a part of this center for healing.

Of all the many experiences I have had in my life, this has been one of the most rewarding.

Dr. Kirk E Mitchell, MD

My personal journey into regenerative medicine began nearly two decades ago when a surgical repair of my right knee, originating from a high school football injury, failed. I was told my knee was "bone-on-bone" and that a knee replacement surgery was my only option by my orthopedic surgeon and radiologist. Somewhat depressed by this prognosis, I was complaining to a client of mine, who recommended an injection procedure as an alternative that his father, a Doctor of Osteopathy, was utilizing to help other patients with similar conditions. With nothing to lose, I hopped a flight from Tampa to Philadelphia and gave it a shot. Long story short, it worked beyond my wildest imagination! I regained my strength and range of motion, and the pain was gone. It still is all these years later.

After this experience, I was not just grateful but also felt compelled to share what I had learned with others—that surgery isn't your only option, and a better alternative exists. So, I convinced the doctor who had injected my knee to open a model clinic with the sole focus of developing and offering non-surgical alternatives for osteoarthritis of the knee and other degenerative joints. It is in that clinic that *The Advanced Arthritis Relief Protocol*™ was born. I'm proud to report that we have trained and certified over 200 privately-owned facilities in 38 states in this procedure. These clinics have successfully treated thousands of patients. One of these clinics, Advanced Regenerative Medicine was founded by the author of this book, Dr. Jeff Selano.

I was lucky enough to meet Dr. Jeff Selano through a mutual acquaintance, and it took no time at all to recognize his passion for healthcare and strong work ethic. These traits led Dr. Selano to abandon his peaceful retirement, sell his beloved Tesla Model S for seed money, and bet his entire retirement fund on the chance that he could build a successful regenerative medical practice. His dream was to offer hope and help to those currently suffering in pain and being told their only options were to either learn to live with the pain for the rest of their life or to go under the knife for costly and risky surgical procedures.

Well, the bet paid off! Not only was Dr. Selano able to open his dream clinic in Centennial, Colorado, but along the way, he learned more than he ever dreamt possible about the field of regenerative medicine and the various treatment alternatives that modern medicine has yielded. That said, he found that many of the patients he came to know and care for through his practice had been horribly misinformed about the topic—often by their own doctors, who had failed to provide a previous solution to their pain. Appalled by how little many of his peers knew and by the extreme detriment this caused to his patients' ability to make informed decisions about their healthcare and bodies, Dr. Selano committed to set the record straight by sharing his experience—and so *End Knee Pain Forever!* came to be!

Please join Dr. Selano on a firsthand account of many of the misconceptions his patients have had and the research and evidence compiled to clear up the various rumors and myths about the regenerative medicine process-what they are, how it works, and if it may be able to help you avoid surgery, relieve your pain, and return to a healthy active lifestyle once more!

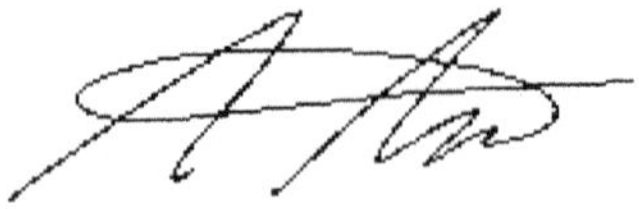

Lance Liberti, MBA

Founder & CEO

Integrative Practice Solutions, LLC

Acknowledgements

I must mention the giants of whom I stand on the shoulders. In the regenerative medicine world, I want to express heartfelt thanks to Lance Liberti, owner of Integrative Practice Solutions. I have had the good fortune to travel the world, and in all my adventures, I have never met someone smarter and more passionate than Lance—in any endeavor. He is a walking encyclopedia of information on regenerative medicine. While not a doctor, he possesses the brains and knowledge that go far beyond some of the brightest minds in this profession. A devourer of research papers and someone quick to tell the truth despite what it might cost him, Lance always has your back. In a world of people who put dollars before patients, Lance continually demonstrates that his word, honor, and ethics are beyond reproach. Thank you, Lance, for being someone who provides clarity and integrity in the regenerative world.

To my wife Mary who has stood by my side through thick and thin. The reason why doctors are in large group practices these days is because they have protection in numbers. That's why you feel like a number in those places. The reason I am a sole practitioner like you remember from when you were a kid is because this is the only way I know how to provide the best care possible without the influence of anyone over me telling me how and what to do. That means you get gold standard care from a small office of people, not a franchise, who care deeply and personally about you and your health. Especially the part about getting you free of knee pain and back to normal life. Being a solo practitioner also comes with a lot of heavy burdens and that's where Mary comes in. She has picked me up off the floor more times than I can count, and I love her now as I have loved her for the past 37 years. In fact, more. Mary this would not be possible without you. Thanks for always believing in me.

Chapter 1

What You Need to Know

If you are reading this book, then you likely either have degenerative joint disease or know someone who spends their day in agonizing and debilitating pain because of it. Is this you? Or is it affecting someone you love? Are you suffering in silence because you don't think you have any other options? You've been to the orthopedic doctor, who prescribed pain meds and anti-inflammatory drugs, only providing temporary relief, and typically doing more long-term damage than good. As a doctor who has spent the last 26 years treating osteoarthritis (OA) patients, I felt compelled to write this tell-all book. The time for you to act is now! There are many just like you—the number of Americans and countless tens of millions, maybe even hundreds of millions, of people around the globe who understand your pain. People suffer in silence. Perhaps they don't go to the doctor, or if they have gone, they have decided it's hopeless since the treatment options typically involve pain meds and anti-inflammatory drugs. Well, it's not hopeless. Let me tell you about a treatment option for you that can change your life.

I hate needles—hate them! However, that makes me super-sensitive to what my patients go through and makes me the best person to own a regenerative medicine OA clinic. OA stands for osteoarthritis. You know, your "old pal Arthur," the kind of friend that you would rather not have. Sadly, far too many people in the world have this "friend." In America alone, it is estimated that one in four adults suffer daily with some form of OA. According to Osteoarthritis Action Alliance (1), that represents roughly 54.4 million people and is expected to jump to 70 million by 2040.

How bad is this problem?

Osteoarthritis represents an annual spend of $65 billion in the US on everything from medicines and surgeries to doctor visits and salves. This study also found that absenteeism from work and lost productivity costs employers an estimated $10.3 billion each year. Collectively, this represents an annual wage loss of around $17 billion for American workers.

These good folks are victims of OA, either because of age and time, wear and tear, or perhaps they have secondary OA, which is the result of an existing (old) injury to a particular joint. Here in Colorado, we have an active community of people who ski or hike or run. After many years of this, their bodies experience a significant amount of deterioration—specifically, their joints and knees.

Knees take the brunt of the injury, and over time, that usually translates to problems with the lower back and feet, too. Often, regenerative clinics only treat your knees and ignore these other areas that play a critical role in your gait. Over time, the lower back, hips, and feet will compensate for a bad gait and will start to experience the same deterioration as the knees. Our job is to arrest that progression and even reverse it, if possible.

> ***"I had no idea the issue with bad knees and joints was this involved until I came to Advanced Regenerative Medicine. What an eye-opener—both with my understanding of how this worked, but also with how it applied to my own body."***
>
> ***-Karen W., Loveland, CO***

How much pressure is put on the knees, on average?

Experts maintain that for every pound of body weight, your knees feel 1.5 pounds of pressure. So, for a standard adult male who weighs 200 pounds, that means up to 300 pounds of pressure is put on the knees, according to a Harvard study (2). That is an incredible amount of weight on two joints of the body. Multiply that by the average amount of steps that someone takes per day—let's say 5000—and you can see how the pounding on your knees really adds up. All the weight-bearing joints share the load to some degree, but the knees take it hardest.

The numbers corresponding to how many people have OA take into consideration the entire body. Someone might have OA in their elbow or shoulder. Perhaps, someone has OA in their hips, lower back, neck, or feet. For the purposes of this book, we focus mainly on the knees, but regenerative therapy works on them all. According to arthritis.org (3), it is estimated that between 2004–2014, around 64% of the patients diagnosed with arthritis by a doctor were younger than 65! Again, from my experience, I say that the percentage is higher than that. So that means we have a two-fold problem. The first is that we want people to be healthy and active. The second is that after years of overdoing it, we have a massive population of people who are headed for total knee replacements…or so they think. Let's talk about that.

> ***"I had heard that your body weight contributed to the deterioration of your knees, but I had no idea how much until I came to Advanced Regen Med. The education has meant as much to me as the help I'm getting."***
>
> ***-Brian K., Castle Pines, CO***

Total Knee Replacement Surgery

Some people do require a total knee replacement. The *Journal of Bone and Joint Surgery* (4) states that in 2008, there were a total of 615,050 total knee replacements— 134% more than were reported a decade earlier. During that same time, the US population only increased by 11%. That dramatic increase has caused many respected medical journals and many in print media to question the necessity of these procedures. In doing so, they are shedding light on the massive profits and marketing efforts that also rose during those periods by drawing people to hospitals and orthopedic centers to receive this procedure. During that same time, another correlative rise in the incidents of Alzheimer's and dementia in the US occurred. Can putting someone over the age of 50 under general anesthesia cause alterations in the brain to create or aggravate these conditions? We will inspect that in the following chapters.

Our goal for you, or someone you love, is to offer insight and education to help avoid a total knee replacement. HA or PRP Injections can dramatically help joint pain sufferers. We see the effects daily in our patients. So many people who feel hopeless and have lost their zest for life have had a rebirth of sorts with the regenerative therapies we provide. It's so gratifying to watch them get their lives back. We will share some of those success stories with you in this book.

> ***"I literally cannot have any surgeries on my knees due to some health complications. I had nowhere to turn, but I also wasn't aware of the incredible risks associated with a total knee replacement. That's frightening."***
>
> ***-Abraham, R., Golden, CO***

Skepticism

The challenge is that people are skeptical of what they incorrectly see as an "experimental" treatment. Or perhaps they have already been through the regenerative medicine process with an unscrupulous provider and have had little to no results. There is a right way and a wrong way with this treatment, just like anything else. We do not accept every patient unless we passionately believe we can help them. To do that, we review their medical history and take images to see what is going on. We do not lick our finger and hold it up in the air to check what direction the wind is blowing. We do not fly blindly into a diagnosis, treatments, and medical procedures. We want to know what is happening with our patients and create a treatment plan for the best outcome for each individual. My father passed along his good name to me, and I'm not going to sell it for a few gold coins.

In this book, we will explain what it means to be a qualified candidate for regenerative therapy. There is little guesswork, if any, when it comes to this. It is illegal to make any guarantees to patients; we simply strive to be transparent and subjectively and objectively evaluate why we think we can help you or someone you love—or not.

> ***"You read so much junk on the internet about lots of things, you don't know who to believe anymore. Dr. Selano and staff took the time to educate me and my wife so that we could make a clear, informed decision before we decided to do this. No other doctor's office***

we looked at did this to the detail that this office did. We are so thankful for that. It matters when people care."

-Maddy and Ashley H., Brighton, CO

My Personal Stake

As I mentioned before, I have been treating patients in the OA world for 26 years. My staff also comes with an incredibly rich and varied background. Personally I am the only owner and that means "The buck stops here". As I mentioned in the forward while thanking my wife, Mary, we have put our whole life savings into this business. That's how much I believe in it. We don't gamble with our own health, and we surely will not gamble with yours. Be incredibly careful when choosing a clinic to do this kind of work. Medical doctors have no limitation of scope in all 50 states, so that means they can take a weekend course and throw up a shingle Monday morning.

My personal stake in this comes from watching my own mother suffer through knee problems related to OA. She is the most active and healthiest senior I have ever known. As time went by, her ability to stay active was compromised and, being a progressive kind of gal, she turned to a regenerative clinic. The distance was too far for her to come to us, but as you can imagine, I watched her progress like a hawk. The turnaround was stunning. Now, none of us can keep up with her and she is 80! She followed the pre-care and post-care protocols religiously and ate very well, including the necessary collagen supplements that are required to build healthy cartilage cells.

Many of our patients so badly want to get better and to ***avoid a total knee replacement***, but they are afraid. I can tell you this unequivocally: You can do this. The process is relatively simple. There is no downtime or recovery time. Weigh that against total knee replacement. Our staff are experts in this field and are also very caring and compassionate. Many folks who are deathly afraid of needles come in and literally walk out, asking, "Was that it?" We take extra measures to ensure your comfort so that the process is enjoyable. And remember, that is coming from the guy who hates needles!

Our Goal for You.

Ultimately, our goal is to help you live your best life. Right now! On average, every day approximately 10,000 people turn 65 (6). This is the largest age demographic in the country—the baby boomers. You have worked hard, and now you have bad knees to show for it. The time for wondering and questioning is over. Act now and get back to the things you love. Medicare loves this. That's right, Medicare actually pays for the hyaluronic injections and knee and special bracing required to ensure your best shot at getting out of knee pain and back to your normal life. So, what are you waiting for? It takes an act of congress to get Medicare to reimburse for anything, so you know the science is sound.

General Anesthesia

Earlier, I mentioned the risks of putting someone out cold for surgery and the potential ramifications that can happen to your brain if you are over the age of 60. According to *International*

Journal Anesthesia (6), there is a connection between midlife exposure to anesthesia and Alzheimer's disease. Yes, you read that right. Is it worth the risk if there is another option to total knee replacement? The study suggests that, in fact, exposure to general anesthetics prior to the age of 50, when your brain is much healthier, can also have a correlative effect on Alzheimer's. Some conditions leave no choice but general anesthesia for treatment or surgery, but when there's another option, why not try?

Statistics

Here are some stats that you're unlikely to hear from your surgeon. According to the highly respected *British Medical Journal* (7), a total knee replacement had "minimal effect on quality of life," especially for patients with severe conditions. This is a stunning finding. Research suggests that up to one-third of those who have had TKR continue to experience chronic pain and that one in five patients, or 20%, are completely dissatisfied with the outcome. The *Washington Post* (8) reports that 33% of patients may not even be appropriate candidates for total knee replacement surgery because their arthritis symptoms are not severe enough to merit the procedure.

Americans are aging and getting heavier, which certainly contributes to the rise in these amputation procedures, but that alone doesn't explain the explosive stats over the past couple of decades. Rates of TKR doubled between 1999–2008, and it is expected that by the year 2030, surgeons will perform 3.5 million of them annually. It's big money for hospitals and doctors who have high overheads and boat payments to make. Not all doctors and hospitals are unscrupulous, of course, but doctors tend to follow the money.

And what about revision surgery for your knees? Can you imagine going through that once, but twice? The failure rate is shocking. It should also be mentioned that there were other complications, ranging from debilitating to life-threatening, in TKR patients who suggested that their procedure helped them with some pain. Consider these other risk factors: blood clots, infection, and severe knee stiffness, causing another surgery and general anesthesia again. And here's the kicker: According to the prestigious *Journal of Bone and Joint Surgery* (9), one out of 100–200 patients who undergo TKR die within 90 days of the procedure. Die! Let that sink in for a moment.

So, to be clear, if having to undergo general anesthesia is absolutely necessary, then the benefits will likely outweigh the risks. I'm referring to medically necessary surgeries that save your life. But knee replacement surgery? You will be told that it must happen and that there is no other option. After finishing this book, you will no longer be able to say that you were not aware that another option existed. An option that is far less invasive and dangerous, has far less downtime, and no rehabilitative or convalescence connected to it. A procedure that allows you to get your life back quickly, help you become active again, and enjoy all the related health benefits connected to that. Living your life vibrantly, to the fullest.

I know you want to get to the good stuff, so let's move on. Next, we will discuss the protocols for what makes you a qualified candidate. We will also discuss the treatment itself, what to expect, and the truths and myths about regenerative medicine. There is a LOT of misinformation out there, and we intend to set the record straight, once and for all. So, come along for this ride with us. I promise you will come away far more educated and informed than you could possibly have imagined. Let's go!

Questions you should ask:

1) What is OA?
2) How much of a problem is OA in America?
3) What effect does body weight have on your knees?
4) What are the real risks of TKR (Total Knee Replacement)
5) What are the real risks of General Anesthesia over the age of 60
6) Is there hope for you?

Chapter 2

Truths and Myths

Regenerative medicine has many myths. We hear daily from patients who have been provided bad information that's presented as actual scientific facts. I'm blown away by the things patients say to us. The misinformation that we regularly hear from our patients is one of the driving forces behind creating this book. Like any technology or medical procedure, the rumor mill starts flying. Doctors with less than good intent tend to jump into that space and fill the void with their own pseudoscience, leading to distrust and confusion as patients are left to navigate what appears to them to be the Wild West. Well, buckle up. Here we will share with you some of the crazy claims that we have heard. You need to know what's true and what's not.

Let's start with the Myths:

1) Regenerative Medicine is experimental. Not true. Research has been going on for over 50 years with volumes of solid double blind medically indexed research behind it. I mentioned earlier that it takes an act of congress to get Medicare to approve anything. While that is frustrating for the people trying to get their treatment protocols vetted, its an important process that Medicare goes through, and it should be done slowly. They want to look at all the white papers and vet all the ins and outs to make sure that its legit. So, when Medicare finally puts their stamp on something you know it's the real deal folks.

2) I can't afford this. Not true. Since Medicare put their stamp on the use of Hyaluronic Acid injections in people with painful knees your policy should cover it. In fact, we are often surprised when we come across an odd, remote policy that doesn't. Truthfully 99.9% of al the insurances for people over the age of 65 that we do a benefits authorization on come back with approvals for all the codes we use. And even those very rare times that it doesn't it usually just takes a quick call from the patient, and we get the approval. All commercial insurances are supposed to follow Medicare's guidelines and pretty much all of them do. As of right now Kaiser Permanente is the only one who flat our refuses. In fact, if you have Kaiser, you can only go to a Kaiser facility to get any care. You can't wander off their reservation. That's how they control the process over you. Other than

that, you are home free. If by chance you happen to have Kaiser it doesn't mean, we can't help you. We have fantastic payment plans that are very affordable. We have never turned anyone away because of money.

3) Medicare won't cover the braces/rehab equipment. Also, NOT true. Part of the rehabilitation process is the durable medical equipment bracing we provide. This is the best way to ensure that you have the greatest chance as a successful recovery from knee pain. There are 3 types of bracing we use, and each plays a very important supportive role. Medicare has created specific codes for each of them after years of study to ensure their efficacy and importance. The knee braces play 2 important roles; the first is to properly align the femur (thigh) bone on the tibia (calf) bone. After years of suffering with increasing knee pain the cartilage starts to deteriorate and usually on the inside of the knee first. As a result, people start becoming "knock kneed" as they call it. Medically this is called Genu Valgus. Even if it's slight, the progressive process can be devastating to the knee, accelerating you into further osteo arthritis. The other important thing the knee braces do is called unloading. The braces are specifically designed to help create space between the bones in your knee that are getting closer and closer to one another causing terrific pain. By holding those slightly open it helps relieve the pain and allows for the space required for the material we inject into your knees to do its work. The take home rehab device we provide you allows you to do your PT at home and not have to come in

for 20 additional visits. This device is very simple to use and is called a static flexion/extension device. Contracture of the knee capsule is present in almost 100% of patients with OA and its very important to get your knee to either full extension or flexion or both. This device also helps move the material we inject across all the different surfaces of your knee for proper distribution. Especially up behind your kneecap where there is also cartilage that is deteriorating. And again, the best part is you get to do this daily in the comfort of your own home. The total time you will use this device is about 10 min per day, twice a day. Easy. Finally, the people upstairs at the federal government did something right. Lastly, and just as important is the back/hip brace. Most of the people we examine either have back pain or pelvic muscle dysfunction resulting in imbalance in their hips. That immediately translates down to the knees as imbalance which has been contributing to their deterioration. This is an extreme example but imagine if for a week you had one heel of your shoe was half an inch thicker than the other. Your knees would throb after only a few days of walking around like that. When we examine our patients on the initial, risk free consultation we find that an unlevel pelvis, with or without pain, has a leg length discrepancy of at least half an inch. So, the reverse of this is simple; use the back brace to level the hips and get the uneven weight distribution off the knees. Without this you will be walking around putting a pounding on one knee and favoring the other and possibly undo all the great work that we are doing to help your knees. We ALWAYS do a complete insurance verification and authorization before we issue these, so you know confidentially that your insurance has approved them for your care plan.

4) I must keep doing this forever. The answer to this fall into a couple of different categories or explanations. Surely if you have OA that is affecting your activities of daily living (ADL) and causing you're a fair amount of pain you are then heading down the road to a total knee replacement at some juncture. Maybe not tomorrow, maybe not next year, but eventually depending on the severity. That is what we and Medicare are trying to prevent. Medicare will allow you to go back through the process every 6 months. That's how much they believe in it. Each round of injections the small glands in your knees that produce hyaluronic acid (the main components of synovial fluid) get stimulated into producing more on your own. Hyaluronic acid works to lubricate your joints all over your body. The problem is that after the age of 45 we tend to make less of it and what we do make is watery thin and not the right thickness to be as effective anymore. So as a result, over time the space between our knees starts to get close and eventually the protective cartilage starts to touch and rub and deteriorate. In theory what we like to see is that you will lose one medical device each time you go through it. If you are in a walker, then you end up with a cane. Then you lose the cane and can walk on your own weight without assistance. Then you can get back to your normal activities. Depending on where you are in that chain it can take one round or multiple rounds. Studies have shown that a minimum of 4 rounds

of injections provides the best results for stimulating your own hyaluronic acid fluid in your knees. And the best part is that if you find it helps you a lot, which most of our patients do, you can avoid the total knee replacement surgery forever if you follow the protocol. Many of our patients come in in the spring and get a round of injections so they can enjoy their summer activities. Golf, walking, pickle ball, softball, hiking, shopping, etc. Then they come back in the fall and do it again so they can get through the winter months until the spring rolls around again. Fantastic. If you were a diabetic and you found that metformin or insulin work, why would you stop the treatment that is working? Make sense?

5) If I have bone on bone this treatment won't work. Categorically untrue. We see many people who claim to be "bone on bone", or worse have been told by their orthopedic surgeon that they are. If I had a nickel for every patient who swears they are bone on bone until we show them their x rays that they are not, I would be Rockefeller. The point is that if you are bone on bone or close to it, we can still help. The unloading knee brace does Its finest work in these situations. By using the knee brace, we create enough space to get the material into the knees and create separation of the degenerative joint surfaces. We see people every month in this condition and with rare exception they get much better.

6) I must wear my braces _all day_. No, that is not true. In fact, I would prefer if you didn't wear them continuously. The knee braces are to be worn, while on your feet, 4 hours a day for 4 months. You can wear them under your clothes. They are very light and not bulky like knee braces from the days gone by. Technology has come quite a long way. To be clear, wearing them while not on your feet does nothing for you so please wear them while weight baring. If you can only wear them an hour or 2 per day for each knee, that's still better than nothing. Anything here is better than what you were doing before, right? The back brace is super important and can be worn while on your feet for the same amount of time. It also is very light and not bulky and can easily be worn under your clothes. We have worked very hard, scouring the land to provide you with the best technology available while staying within Medicare's strict guidelines. These are not off the shelf, CVS,Walmart or Walgreens braces. Not even close. These are specially manufactured and approved devices per Medicare's standards.

7) This treatment does not regrow my knee cartilage. While the treatment itself does not regrow the cartilage, your body is always attempting to do that for you. Even as you sit here and read this book your body is trying to repair it. That process will never stop until you breathe your last. The problem of OA is that as the gap between your knees gets closer and closer and the cartilage is pressing down harder and harder, the blood supply to it is getting suffocated.

Which, like a tornado, keeps the process spinning out of control. By injecting hyaluronic acid (also sometimes known in medical circles as Viscosupplementation) along with the knee braces we create the space between your knees to allow your own body to start to repair the cartilage. This is evident when we do our post treatment follow ups at 90 days and 6 months where we take images again to see what progress has been made. The worse off you are when you start the slower the progress, but progress is being made none the less. So it's better to start as soon as you can instead of waiting and letting it get worse.

8) You should only do one knee at a time. That is only true if you have had a total knee replacement on one of those knees. We will discuss this more in the following chapter under the section called Bilateral knees. One knee is usually in trouble and since the pain is aggressive it easy to focus on that knee and think the other is "fine". Most of the time the knee that is "fine" is in trouble too. Just not as aggressively. Usually, a grade 2 on the Kellengren-Lawrence scale where 4 is bad and 1 is very mild. Getting in front of the knee that is "fine" is always the best course of action so that we can stop it from getting as bad as the one that is killing you. Of course, we must do our due diligence and test that other knee to see if it fits the strict Medicare requirements for treatment. More on that in the next chapter.

Things you should understand.

1) The importance of bracing and why.
2) The importance of hyaluronic acid in the knee and what it does.
3) Does this work if I'm bone on bone?
4) The reasons for daily use of the braces.
5) Can the cartilage in my knees regrow?
6) Why its important to do both knees.

Chapter 3

Who Qualifies and Why?

Patient Qualifications

We do not accept all patients. Sometimes that comes as a shock to people because, in our capitalistic, free marketplace environment, patients often think that healthcare is like Burger King, "have it your way"; they get to pick and choose. While this is true to some extent, at the end of the day, we decide whether we want to accept the patient or not based on subjective and objective evidence. After all, the patient does not pay my malpractice insurance. Most patients do not look at medicine this way, but we want to be certain that we have vetted all possible factors to make a reasonable and responsible decision on your care.

I never know what insurance a patient has. Never have. I do not want to know, if I am being completely honest. I do not ever want to be influenced by that information. The truest and most honest way to practice medicine is to advise the patient on what treatment is going to be best for them, regardless of what they can or cannot afford. I do not even know if an existing patient owes me money or not. Again, I do not want to be influenced by that information either. While that might seem Pollyanna-ish for some people, it is the only way I know how to run a responsible and effective practice. It has probably cost me a fortune over 26 years, but I do not care. It is honest and upholds the good name my parents taught me to protect.

So, when a patient reaches out to us, the first thing we do is gather the information we can from them. Things like their health history, any medications or surgeries they have had. Especially if they have tried and failed any conservative treatments like cortisone shots or PT or over the counter pain relievers. Most people have done these things before they come to us. Many have tried to lose weight too, but we all know how that goes. We have the best of intentions, but the weight usually doesn't come off or it does and then comes back.

One thing I have subscribed to in my 30 years in practice is this; Healing begins with that first point of contact, not with my medical staff or me. We all have better things to do than just make a random phone call to a doctor's office, right? The people who call us have already decided that they have some level of interest, and based on how we answer their questions, they will decide if they want to move on to the next phase to the no cost, no risk consultation. The next step is to make an initial appointment. However, this will never happen if the person on the phone makes the patient feel like they are insignificant in any way. We are blessed to have an amazing and caring staff who understand that making the patient feel welcomed is crucial. They need to feel that we are invested in their healing. Sadly, not all doctor's offices are like that. We will never deviate from this. Remember, we are patients too and we treat you the way we want to be treated when we go to the doctor.

Preparation

Once we have scheduled an appointment, we prepare for that first important day with them. When they arrive, we have them complete and sign all the necessary paperwork and take them to the imaging room. Here, we take static images of their knees. Both AP (anterior-posterior) and lateral (side) so that we can accurately see what is going on. There is a grading scale for the condition of their knees that goes from grade 1–4. This is called the Kellengren-Lawrence scale for Osteo Arthritis. Grade 1 is the best and grade 4 is the worst. Grade 4 is what most people are referring to when they say "bone-on-bone." However, even in grade 4 cases, there is still some cartilage in there. Maybe not much cartilage, but enough to go to work. Often in grade 2, 3 and 4 cases, we see erosion and loss of space between the bones along with bones spurs starting to grow. We often see that the space behind the kneecap is getting smaller and smaller. There is cartilage behind your knees and that allows it to slide back and forth across the bottom of your femur. In fact, in the grand design, there is a groove at the bottom of your femur where your kneecap glides. When we run our range of motion and orthopedic tests, we often feel grinding or "clicking" with pain when we test the knee cap. This is a clear sign of something called "chondromalacia patella". Fancy medial talk for the cartilage behind your kneecap that is deteriorating.

When I went through gross anatomy the body that we worked on had this. When we lifted back the knee cap the bottom of it looked like what an apple looks like when you cut it and leave it out on the counter for a few hours. Brown and rotted and pitted with holes. The good news is that the hyaluronic acid we inject is allowed to flow up behind the kneecap as well and create some space there too. This allows your body to start the repair process with that cartilage along with the joint space between your knees. Therefore, we always using fluoroscopy when we do injections. We never guess. For the material to get where it's supposed to be we MUST see where we are going. There are too many ways you can miss, and we never miss. Too many providers in this business just roll up your pant leg, give you a shot in the knee, pat you on the head and call it good. That's garbage medicine and its incredibly irresponsible in my humble opinion.

Often, the turning point is when the patient actually sees the images. This helps them understand the importance of the treatment. Many patients have told us that one of their knees is either fine or that it is giving them some mild discomfort while the other is intensely painful. What they don't realize is that both knees are usually in trouble, but the one that is giving them the most grief is outweighing the sensory output of the other. For instance, if you have a big toe on your left foot that is hot, swollen, and painful, it will draw most of your focus. If you have a big toe on the right side that is also bothering you, you most likely won't pay much attention to that side. The same thing seems to happen with knee joints. In medicine, this is often referred to as cortical distraction. It simply means that the condition that is yelling the loudest (most painful) draws most of your attention.

Bilateral Knee Issues

It is rare for the less painful knee to not have any state of deterioration, which as you now know we call OA or osteo arthritis. I have only seen one case where the other knee was actually fine when the other was a mess. When you start to compensate for your bad knee, you alter your lower back, your feet, and thus your entire gait. Recall when I mentioned how many times you take steps every day on average? Well, imagine years of that altered gait and how much compensatory damage is taking place on the "non-involved" joints elsewhere. I have even witnessed problems in a patient's upper back and neck due to this process.

Think of it this way: If the bottom of the Empire State Building was tilted by a degree, the top would hang over by 20 feet. In your body, when your lower framework is just slightly out of alignment, it translates all the way up to your head. At our clinic, we endeavor to treat people as a whole person and not just a collection of parts. So, if there are significant issues with just one knee, over time it will have an adverse effect on the rest of your locomotion. Over time, it will affect the alignment of every other part of your body.

If the other knee is experiencing a grade 2 or worse, then we typically recommend treating both knees. This is the best-case scenario because the quicker you can get in front of the problem, the better the outcome typically is. And let's face it—the other knee is going down the same tracks as the more painful one, and then you'll just have to do it all over again. Plus, it's better to heal bilaterally than unilaterally (one side) as far as joint health is concerned.

The Examination

Next, we do a knee examination that involves palpation and testing range of motion combined with some orthopedic tests to see if we can confirm what we have found on the images. This is usually not as powerful for the patient as seeing the images, but it is clinically important, if not critical, to come up with a final assessment. When evaluating the complete health history, we greatly consider the medications the patient is taking. For instance, we look at blood thinners and blood pressure or diabetes medications. We evaluate all medications or conditions that might influence the patient's ability to heal. There are no rejections with our various treatments, and they do not adversely affect or react with any prescription medications.

As with any injection, there is always the chance that someone can experience side effects, ranging from infection to mild swelling, tenderness, and some mild discomfort at the injection site. We take all the proper steps to mitigate these presentations. If someone is on high doses of blood thinners, that does not mean they cannot proceed with the procedure, but our medical staff will advise them on what to expect. While coumadin and warfarin are still in use, they are prescribed less frequently these days. Still, if you are taking blood thinners, our medical staff will want to be in communication with your primary doctor to get their input and see that your INR (international normalized ratio), a measure of how well your body can form clots, is low enough to allow us to proceed.

The Two Main Treatment Options

Now that we have all your pertinent medical information, we will decide if we want to recommend a course of treatment based on our findings. If we feel it is safe to proceed and the patient agrees, we will set up a time for their first treatment. We offer two versions: ***PRP (platelet-rich plasma), or hyaluronic gel injections***. We might recommend a combination of these if we feel that would best serve the patient. Only an experienced practitioner will know how to combine these, so ensure you ask about their experience. In this case we will do the hyaluronic Acid (HA) injections first and then do the PRP. We don't do them simultaneously. Its too much for the knee to deal with all at the same time. Lets do one thing very well and then move on to the next thing.

PRP Injections

The second treatment option is PRP. PRP, or platelet-rich plasma, is a procedure where we draw the patient's blood, spin it in a centrifuge, and then draw out the yellow plasma into a separate syringe. According to Johns Hopkins, PRP is not only chock-full of concentrated platelets and growth factors but also helpful proteins that facilitate and trigger cell proliferation. This aids in accelerating healing and stimulates tissue regeneration. Patients respond very well to these injections, which are typically given in a series of three scheduled a month apart. Since PRP comes from your own body, it is the most popular treatment option.

PRP injections will result in the same regenerative growth of the damaged joint tissues that allografts will produce. However, PRP does take longer for the body to regrow the tissues, but it produces stunning results. Many professional athletes' careers have been saved by PRP, from Peyton Manning, Hines Ward, Tiger Woods, and beyond. After we draw out the PRP, we place it into a bio-incubator. This heats up the sample and begins an important process called the thrombin (or clotting) cascade. This is crucial for the concentrated PRP to coagulate, and it helps facilitate a greater healing process. By warming it up and turning it into a gel, it will also last a lot longer in the joint, like an extended-release tablet your PCP might prescribe. The longer we can keep it in the joint, the better your outcomes will be.

Hyaluronic Acid Gel Injections

Sometimes referred to as "gel shots". The reason for this pseudonym is that proper HA should be thicker than water, have more density. The type we use is called Genvisc 850. It is the same molecular weight as the kind of HA your body makes naturally. The only contraindications as follows. *CONTRAINDICATIONS Do not administer to patients with known hypersensitivity (allergy) to sodium hyaluronate preparations. Do not inject this product in the knees of patients with infections or skin diseases in the area of the injection site.* That literally comes right off the manufacturers website. Compared to just about everything else that you can be prescribed that comes with 2 full pages, single lines of things that can go wrong, you can see that this is pretty inert. Lets take them one at a time. Allergy to sodium hyaluronate preparations. What does this mean?

To keep it relatively straightforward I'll put it this way. HA is used globally in skin treatments for men and women. They are used 90% of the time by women and only 10% by men according to reports. If you have used anything like this an had any issues you should put that on your history form. That doesn't mean we won't be able to proceed but would involve asking more questions about your experience. The fact is we make HA naturally in our own bodies and the amount we are putting into your knee capsule is small. Then you have to consider the fact that its contained in your knee capsule and doesn't spread throughout your body. So it's incredibly safe and to be honest we have never once had anyone have any reaction to it because of these facts. Not one person. Compare that to the long list of problems that an aspirin can cause and we all take those from time to time without ever reading the list of contraindications provided. Still, we want to know if by some remote chance you have had any issues with it before then we will investigate further.

Hyaluronic acid is the primary component of synovial fluid, which is in every joint in the human body. Think of it like oil—it is what gives the joint the ability to move without creaking or grinding. Remember when Dorothy put oil in the Tin Man's joints? Same thing. Over time, we produce less and less HA, and as a result, the capsule in your knee loses height, like a tire going flat. Eventually, the bones get closer and closer and the deterioration is agonizing for most. To perform this procedure, we need to see that the gel is actually going directly into the joint capsule. No guessing.

HA Gel injections do not regrow any tissue. They help separate the joint spaces, much like inflating a tire, and offer some pain relief. Many patients come to see us in the spring when softball season begins because they haven't done much all winter and need a tune-up. The injection will last for a few months, and then they are usually back in the fall to do it again. HA gel injections should be given in a series of five, spaced a week apart. If we do these bilaterally, then we typically will do the left knee on a Tuesday and the right knee on a Thursday.

Why Is Imaging Important?

For imaging, we use our fluoroscopy machine for all procedures to make sure we are in the correct location. In fact, we use our imaging machine on all injections, regardless of the substance we are using. Doing these types of injections under imaging is critical. I'm stunned when a patient tells us that their previous provider just rolled up their pant leg and did a blind injection. Yikes. How do you know you are in the right location? How do you know you are not in a fat pad or the bursa or behind the kneecap? When I bring this up with other practitioners, the typical response goes something like this: "I have been doing this a long time. I know what I'm doing and where I'm going." Hmmmm. Maybe that's why they are now in my office, unhappy with their previous results.

Imaging is so important that we will not do a procedure without it. In the next chapter, we are going to explain the entire process to you. After you read how it's supposed to be done, I'm confident that you'll never let anyone do a knee injection without imaging again. In fact, Medicare requires it. And the procedure shouldn't be done with ultrasound, either. For large joint injections, you need to use fluoroscopy. That is a recent major change that you should be aware of. If anyone in a regenerative clinic comes at you with a needle and they are not using imaging to see where they are going, run!

Questions you should ask:

1) Do all patients qualify for these regenerative treatments?
2) What are the different grades of knee degeneration?
3) Why should I be concerned about the (supposedly) non-involved knee?
4) What are the two main types of regenerative treatment options for me?
5) Why is imaging crucial?

Chapter 4

The Procedure

On the day of the procedure, our medical staff will get everything set up for you. Everything is sterile and sanitized. The trays and equipment are all prepped and ready for each patient. In the morning, before any patients arrive, we have our morning meeting and go through each patient we are going to see that day. We carefully review the procedures we are going to do and any special considerations we need to be aware of. When the patients enter the room, the medical staff will greet them with a warm welcome and a reassuring smile. They get on the table, and we move the fluoroscopy machine into place around their knee. If the weather is nice, we encourage them to wear shorts on injection day to make it easier for them and our staff to have direct access to their knee. However, it's not a problem to roll up a pant leg or put them in a gown if they prefer, but we typically don't use a gown unless the patient requests it.

The Capsule

Here is a brief lesson on the anatomy of the knee. There is a capsule inside everyone's knee that works like a shock absorber. It is roughly about the size of a deflated tennis ball. The capsule walls are made of a specialized connective tissue that holds a fluid called synovial fluid. All joints in your body have this. Think of synovial fluid as motor oil. It's very slippery and viscous. As we age, we produce less of this fluid, and that becomes a problem. Over time, joints will dry out and get creaky, like the Tin Man from *The Wizard of Oz,* if you will. The main component of synovial fluid is hyaluronic acid, or HA.

That's what the gel is in the capsule—hyaluronic acid. As of this book's writing, we use Genvisc 850, which is the exact molecular weight of actual HA. This is important because we want it to reproduce what you have lost over time. As we mentioned earlier you have glands in your knees that make HA for you, but as you age you tend to make less than required and the consistency is more like a watery substance than the necessary thicker "gel" like substance that you used to make when you were 18. Getting older sucks. I get it. However, there is no need to succumb anymore to the aging affects that hinder your happiness.

Another cool component of using this HA product is that, over time, it can actually teach or train your knees to start making HA again. And lastly, it's in gel form. That's critical because the HA you make when you get older is watery and thin. No good. We want to replenish the kind of HA that you made when you were 18—not watery, not thin, but a gel-like consistency that provides a fantastic buffer for your joints. So, to this end, we basically "re-inflate" the tire and pump that joint space back open. It doesn't hurt at all, but you might feel some pressure for a day or so because we have just filled the balloon back up. Make sense? Awesome. Let's move forward.

How We Prepare

We sterilize the injection site thoroughly with Chloroprep and position the needle beside the knee. Then, we take an image to ensure we are in the right location. This allows us to adjust the injection site if needed before putting the needle in their knee. Patients greatly appreciate that. We use a freezing spray called ethyl chloride to numb the injection site and then insert the needle. Patients rarely feel anything. Lidocaine is in the first syringe, which we inject and then advance the needle into that numbed area. We repeat that process until we are in the capsule. Again, it's rare that patients describe any discomfort. If anything, they may experience some mild burning from the lido, but that subsides almost instantly.

Don't Miss

The image during the procedure is critical to ensure the right location is obtained. Then, we insert dye and watch it flow into the capsule space. We start the fluoroscopy machine's video function and take a movie of the dye flowing into the joint capsule. By doing this, we are absolutely sure we are in the right location. If not, this is the time to reposition the needle and insert more dye. While this might sound complicated, it actually isn't for trained staff like mine. One thing to be mindful of is that if there is a tear in the capsule, then the dye will squirt out the back or posterior side, like how jelly squirts out of a donut. If we see that, we know it's time to change the treatment regimen. That's a hard stop.

What If We See a Capsule Tear?

If we see a tear, we will stop the process and begin a regimen of physical therapy and nutritional support to help the capsule repair itself. This usually takes three months. After that, we will repeat the process and be certain that we do not see any dye leaking out of the capsule. There is no point proceeding with the gel injection if we see this happen because as soon as you stand up, all the gel with exit the tear. Makes sense, right? Again, how can anyone do these types of knee injections without imaging? It's unconscionable.

Assuming we do not see any tear in the capsule from the dye injection, we then proceed to the final step and insert the proper selected material (HA or PRP). The entire procedure takes less than 10 minutes in the hands of my talented staff and our advanced equipment. Then, we begin the post-care process, and you are on your way. As long as you take it easy on injection day, you aren't really restricted from any activities, aside from using a trampoline or doing jumping jacks. Many people go about their day, playing golf in the afternoon or going shopping. In fact, it's better to do some activity on injection day; don't go home and be a couch potato. Motion is life and life is motion.

Modifications to the Procedure

In the case of PRP injections, we will first draw the patient's blood and then take it to our lab, where we carefully prepare it as mentioned in the previous chapter. This takes an extra 10–15 minutes to be sure we get it right—no rushing!

This chapter is short is because the procedure is short. It literally takes minutes to do the HA procedures.

Questions you should ask:

1) What should I expect on treatment day?
2) Why is it important to have images taken prior to the treatment?
3) Why is it important to do imaging while the procedure is happening?
4) How is PRP Prepared?

Chapter 5

Post Care

Bracing, PT, and homework.

What to Expect

Immediately following the injection, the patient goes through physical therapy, which usually involves pedaling on a stationary bike. This helps to evenly distribute the material inside the knee. If the patient has any soreness, which is rare, we will use an ice pack for a few minutes until that feeling subsides. Many patients share that they experienced a feeling of pressure in their joint afterward. Regardless of the location, whether it be their knee or elbow or shoulder, this is a normal sensation that will last a day or two. It should be expected since we have just filled up your joint with additional fluid. This feeling will go away fairly quickly and does not typically cause any discomfort.

Actually, the sensation assures you that we got the material in the right location.

Homework

It is a well-known fact, and scholars maintain, that patients who participate in their healing do much better and heal faster than patients who don't. It's quite simple—you get out what you put in. And because we are dealing with connective tissue, you must do certain things while you are not here under our watchful eye to provide better outcomes.

Like I mentioned before, we recommend that patients do not go home and lay around the house; it is better if they walk around. Nothing strenuous, of course, but just go about their normal day. We let them know that if they experience any redness, heat, or soreness, it's fine to use an ice pack for 10 minutes at a time at home. Most patients report that they didn't have to do this at all. We ask patients who use blood thinners to carefully watch their joint and let us know if they have any swelling or discomfort. If their INR numbers are low, they should not have any issues with hematomas or swelling. Again, this is where a skilled practitioner can be invaluable because they know how to properly inject a patient on blood thinners to minimize any issues.

Bracing—The How and Why?

Now, we move on to bracing. This is a hugely important step in your full recovery. If you want to maximize your results, then wearing the bracing we prescribe is critical. Our braces do not impede your ability to do anything. People leave our office with them and go about their lives. We use the smallest braces on the market that still provide the maximum unloading benefits, so your knee can have a chance to heal and provide room for tissue growth.

We use specialized unloading knee braces to assist your knee joint in maintaining a degree of separation so that you don't squash your new cells. These are not your run-of-the-mill drugstore braces. They are specialized DME (durable medical equipment), custom-fitted braces that are essential to your progress. Our medical staff is specially certified to prescribe these vital braces. It's critical that you don't use one from your friend, family, or neighbor, or even one that has been prescribed to you before. Because they are custom fitted at the time of your first injection, any previous device is likely to not fit properly as your body contour and gait will have changed over time. We recommend that you wear the knee braces for four hours a day when you are on your feet. If you are home and have your feet up on the couch, you can take them off.

Doing PT at home to help you strengthen and support your knees and the surrounding muscles, tendons and ligaments. This is very important; so many muscles atrophy over time because you compensate for your injury by altering your biomechanics. You will overuse some muscles and underuse others. If you don't build those muscles back up and just regrow new cartilage cells, then you will end up back where you started. Most clinics ignore this part of the treatment, which is sad because it ends up giving us all a bad name. We employ another fantastic DME that you take home with you so you can do your ongoing PT in the comfort of your home. The device is very easy to use at home, very comfortable and can even be done while in bed. Stretching the contracted knee capsule is a very important part of your recovery. Medicare doesn't get a lot of things right, but this one they did. They knew that if you had the chance to do your own PT at home and not have to drive across town and sit for an hour in the waiting room of the PT clinic, you would be more likely not to quit and be more motivated to do it yourself. And they were right. The compliance that our patients demonstrate is remarkable when they can do their PT in their houses on their own schedule each day. Fantastic!

But My Lower Back Doesn't Hurt!

Symptoms are a weird duck. Problems in one part of your body can present as symptoms or damage somewhere else. People having a heart attack feel pain in their left arm. Women with a bad gallbladder often report pain under their right shoulder blade. Patients with a misalignment in their neck often present with numb fingers. If you step on a dog's tail, it barks out the other end. You dig? This custom fitted pelvic DME is not prescribed for back pain, unless you do have back pain (which most of our patients do), it is for supporting weak and unbalanced muscles in your lower back, hips and pelvis. These issues are part of the reason why your knees are in trouble. Hip bone connected to the….Leg bone. We all remember that song. Well it very much applies here. Its called the "kinetic Chain" and its how your gait and lower body movement either works or doesn't work in a symmetrical fashion.

So when evaluating your knees, we want to know if this is a gait anomaly from your lower back or hips, or did your knees throw your back and hips out of alignment? Chicken or the egg? Doesn't really matter as long as we don't help one and completely ignore the other. Patients will often say, "But my lower back doesn't hurt."

We spoke earlier how important this DME is to get your hips level and therefore your legs even so that when you take steps you are not underutilizing one leg and over working the other. This will result in very poor results with your treatment. The Pelvic Brace we use is very specialized and will be custom fitted to your body so that your hips will be level and your gate will be normalized. This results in much quicker recovery or improvement for our patients. Your run of the mill pharmacy lumbar or lower back brace cannot do what ours does and *any outside bracing not prescribed by us and custom fitted by us is not a part of the protocol.*

Do I Have to Eat That?

Nutrition also plays a critical part in your recovery. If you skip this, you will marginalize your results. Why? Your body requires certain ingredients to make new cells. As your knees call out for material to make these new cells, you better have these important ingredients in your pantry—or body. Think of it this way. You can't make a cake out of sand. Well, you can, but you won't make a very good cake. To that end, you can't make a good cell out of a French fry. Your body will still attempt to make one, but the cell walls will be fragile. Think about the little pigs that made a house out of straw. Same concept.

The true miracle of life is that you put food in one end of the tube and it eventually comes out the other end. Somewhere in between, your body will pull out what it needs to keep you alive. It's truly a miracle that we all have lived this long. Your body's number one directive is the survival of the species. So, you can make a heart cell out of a sausage biscuit, but you will pay for it. So, what do you need in the "pantry" to make good cells? For connective tissue, like cartilage, you need collagen. And not just any collagen, you need pharmaceutical-grade collagen. That way, if you are still going to eat junk food, you will at least have the proper ingredients available when your knees call out for it.

Either way, lower back and hip alignment have to be addressed, or you will be back in here six months from now, mad at us for taking your money. There is an easy way to help the patient see the imbalance in their hips. As part of our initial exam, we also evaluate the condition of your pelvic girdle. That's a fancy way of saying that we will take a close look at the condition of your hips and lower back to see if you require a back brace to provide leveling and alignment. This is not your garden variety back brace. Those won't achieve the results we want for you. Let me give you an example of how this works.

We will have you stand on two side-by-side scales to see if you are leaning one way or the other. Let's say you weigh 200 pounds. If your hips and lower back are perfectly aligned, then it stands to reason that you would see 100 pounds on the left scale and 100 pounds on the right. This is almost never the case with people who have bad knees. Understandably, they will be leaning or favoring one side over the other due to pain. When we see this, we place one of these special DME back braces on them and have them get back on the dual scales. Usually, this will offer some form of corrected balance that is easily witnessed on the scales. However, some mild correction is not sufficient. We will then use this special back brace to compensate.

To do this, our specially trained staff can cinch up one side of the brace tighter than the other and assist you in achieving almost perfect balance. This is easy to see on the dual scales. If we can get you within a five-pound difference from one side to the other, then we have mechanically achieved something you would not be capable of on your own. Now, with your hips and lower back aligned, you can regrow connective tissue in your knees in a way that will be bilaterally uniform. You will have a much greater chance of long-term success. We recommend wearing the back brace for four hours a day.

Why Is This Important?

As you can see, the post-care process is very important to get right. If your current or future clinic does not follow these protocols, then you should find one that does. I don't want to take someone's money and then have them come back in six months and be mad at us. I want to give every patient the best possible chance for the greatest success. Now, if you go home and don't use your braces and follow your post-care instructions, that's not on us. If you don't use the nutritional support we have given you, that's not on us. Sadly, some patients don't follow the rules we have presented them. We are not going to follow you around with a camera to be sure. You must play an active role in your recovery and be responsible for your care when you are not with us.

When you come in, we thoroughly explain all of this, so there is no confusion or misunderstanding of the process. We want you to know what success looks like. At the end of the day, we can only advise you, treat you, and show you where the winning lottery ticket is hidden. You have to act on your own behalf and win.

Recipes From the Pantry?

There is a specific recipe for making new connective tissue cells, just like your grandmother had a specific recipe to make your favorite dessert. These "recipes," if you will, have been welded into our DNA since the beginning of time. The recipe doesn't change. Only you can put the right ingredients into your mouth and ensure that you are giving your body the best chance to heal. To that end, we have made a high-level nutritional supplement available to our patients that have all the right ingredients to help you build new and healthy cells based on the patient's biochemistry.

We spoke earlier about how bad knees affect your feet, back, and spine. Back braces are also an important consideration for our specific treatment protocol. If your hips or lower back are out of alignment, which occurs in almost 97% of the cases we see, then to regrow balanced knee cartilage in an even and uniform way, you must address hip and lower back alignment. Most clinics don't consider this important biomechanical fact.

Questions you should ask:

1) What are the braces for, and why do I have to wear them?
2) Why do I have to do homework?
3) Can I get this kind of treatment if I take anything that thins my blood?
4) Why is nutrition so important to my recovery and healing?

Chapter 6

Testimonials From Our Satisfied Clients

You have heard me talk about this subject from the clinical and medical sides, but now I want you to hear from some of our satisfied patients. Their words are powerful as they have received proper education on what we do and why and been through the procedure and post-care process. Enjoy.

"When I first heard about regenerative medicine, I was skeptical. You read and hear things, you know. But I have been very well pleased with my results. When I first arrived, I was using a cane and was having trouble going up and down the stairs. I was even having trouble getting on and off the toilet! At this point, I am five months past my treatment, and I can walk without the use of any aids and I can do most of my daily activities. I would recommend this to anyone who doesn't want a knee replacement."

-Patty R., Centennial, CO

"I love to ski, and over time, my knees took a pounding. I followed my primary doc's instructions and took over-the-counter things, like ibuprofen and Icy Hot. After that didn't work, I started with cortisone shots. I had no idea how that was like pouring gas on a fire. The pain went away for a little while, but it was making my knees worse. When I came in, I couldn't do a deep knee bend and the stairs were hell. I followed all the recommendations because I did not want knee surgery if it could be avoided. Thank God that's all in the past. Now I am able to ski again and I can go up and down the stairs with no issues. So blown away by this regenerative technology. I would tell anyone to do this."

-Paul S., Ft. Collins, CO

"I came in specifically looking for PRP treatment because my sister had it done, and it seemed to help her a lot. The staff was very helpful and explained everything to me so that I could fully understand what it was all about. The procedure was almost 100% pain-free. I couldn't believe it. I loved the idea of using my own plasma in my own body, knowing that it was super concentrated with all the elements and antibodies that were mine alone. At first, I only had trouble with one of my knees, but when I looked at the imaging, I was shocked to see that my other knee was starting to go downhill as well. So, I had both knees done, and now I can walk two miles a day and go shopping without any pain. This is like a miracle!"

-Karen P., Lone Tree, CO

Chapter 7

Finale

I have scoured the earth looking for a book like this, and frankly, it doesn't exist. With this knowledge, you are now armed with education and a proper understanding of how these processes work in both the body and in a clinical treatment setting. From soup to nuts. Be mindful that if someone tells you different, it might reflect the quality of their training, staff, education, etc. There are different levels of understanding in all kinds of businesses regarding the products, their efficacy, the procedures used, and how to derive the best outcomes. In this case, human lives and health are in the balance, so it's crucially important to pick a clinic that will provide you the best opportunity to succeed. You are well aware of this already. Folgers coffee is quite different from high-end drip coffee. The New York Yankees and the Cleveland Mud Hens are not on the same level. We understand that there are comparative quality differences in any profession. Don't you want the best when it comes to your health?

Sadly, as I have stated earlier, many in this field have a strategy to separate you from your wallet, rather than give you quality healthcare. Do they have a boat payment to make this month? Sadly, this is often their motivation. They are cutting corners for some reason. Be mindful of what advice you are getting from other clinics. If they use inferior products, then you should politely excuse yourself and go elsewhere. If they don't use fluoroscopy for their imaging, consider another clinic that does. If they don't put value in at home PT or bracing or nutritional support, you're destined to fail.

Caution!

Now, to be fair, some patients report that they have had some margin of success at a different clinic that does not follow these responsible steps that I have outlined for you. I have to be honest and say that is the exception, not the norm. Please be mindful that if you or a friend or family member have had this experience, it might not represent the larger percentage of customers who have gone down the same road, only to find themselves still in pain and a bit poorer as a result. There's an old Latin saying, "caveat emptor," meaning buyer beware.

If you are not armed with knowledge about what you are buying, then it is definitely hard to make informed decisions. Many are doing it the right way and using ethical practices, but far too many are not. But how are you supposed to know the difference? Well, now you do. What you do with these valuable tools is, of course, up to you. To help you navigate the "Wild West," we have provided valuable questions at the end of each chapter to ask at your first consultation. This will help you determine if you have found the right clinic, based on how they answer these questions.

Take Heart

If you are suffering from joint pain in your knees or other joints, take heart that there is a solution for you that does not involve surgery and all its potential dangers. To that end, there are some people that surgery is their only reasonable option. I know many of them. For some of our patients who have had to go down that road, we take heart in knowing that we helped them achieve healthier joints prior to surgery, which inevitably helped them recover faster and prepared them for an easier surgical experience, even in the case of total knee replacement.

While all of our progress was removed, the time that we were able to help them regain more mobility helped them become more active, which improved their health immensely. Having more mobility helped improve their immune and vascular systems. It helped regain muscle strength and flexibility that they had long since lost due to atrophy and deterioration. In that way, a course of regenerative treatment should not only be considered prior to surgery but should be mandatory. Taking someone who has an overall unhealthy body from lack of motion and mobility and cutting off their knees is a recipe that leads to a very difficult recovery period and sometimes convalescence, or even death.

So, even if you or someone you love is being told that a total knee replacement is their only option, you should consider the immense benefits of a course of regenerative therapy beforehand to give you the best chance of moving forward. Literally. It's not about how many years in your life, but how much life you can put into your years. You have busted your tail all your life, and you want to live it to the fullest and enjoy the remaining years you have in the best possible health. When it comes to people with bad knees and joints, now you know how to do that.

Hopefulness

While it's so important to provide the warnings and the cautions, we also want to share the positive side with you. Pain is a funny thing. Some people have pain, and some people are a pain. There is a difference. We have all spent many collective decades in the pain world here at Advanced Regenerative Medicine, and we try our best to understand that difference. Pain sucks—let's face it. It can make a rough day worse. However, the antidote is hope. The worst feeling is that of hopelessness. If you are in pain and don't have options, it's easy to lose faith. We want to assure you that there are better days ahead for you. There is light at the end of the tunnel, and it's not an oncoming train. No matter your ADL (activities of daily living) goals, we are here to help you achieve them. For some, it's simply living without pain. For others, it might be the ability to get on the carpet once again and play with their grandkids. I know that many people tell us that they are excited to just go for a walk or play golf or go shopping again without the pain. There is hope, but you must find the right provider who can answer all your questions the right way. There is hope because now you are armed with the knowledge you need to vet the doctors and staff who have your best interests, and not their pocketbook, at heart. So, get out there and take the bull by the proverbial horns, do the research, ask the right questions, and live your best life!

Our clinic is in Centennial, CO. Please come in and see us. We will be happy to do a no-obligation consultation to help determine if this is the right treatment for you.

Colorado Knee and Spine Clinic/
Advanced Regenerative Medicine

6726 S. Revere Pkwy STE 180

Centennial, CO 80112

720-681-6170

www.advregenmed.com

References

Gonzalez study

https://www.bayoaksphysicalmed.com/wp-content/uploads/2018/04/Stem-cell-Gonzalez-3rd-party-testing-White-Paper.pdf

Referenced Studies

1 Osteoarthritis Action Alliance

https://oaaction.unc.edu/oa-module/oa-prevalence-and-burden/

2 Harvard study

https://www.health.harvard.edu/pain/why-weight-matters-when-it-comes-to-joint-pain

3 Arthritis.org

https://www.arthritis.org/getmedia/e1256607-fa87-4593-aa8a-8db4f291072a/2019-abtn-final-march-2019.pdf

4 Journal of Bone and Joint Surgery

https://journals.lww.com/jbjsjournal/Abstract/2012/02010/The_Dramatic_Increase_in_Total_Knee_Replacement.2.aspx

5 US Census

https://www.census.gov/library/stories/2019/12/by-2030-all-baby-boomers-will-be-age-65-or-older.html

6 Journal of Anesthesia

https://www.ncbi.nlm.nih.gov/pmc/articles/PMC6443620/

7 British Medical Journal

https://www.bmj.com/content/356/bmj.j1131

8 Washington Post

https://www.washingtonpost.com/national/health-science/treatment-or-torment-some-knee-replacements-fail-to-solve-chronic-pain/2018/12/21/76d5aa42-ffe6-11e8-862a-b6a6f3ce8199_story.html

9 Journal of Bone and Joint Surgery

https://www.ncbi.nlm.nih.gov/pubmed/28375889

Made in the USA
Monee, IL
20 April 2022

95055280R10036